I0441679

The Insulin Resistance Diet

The Ultimate Guide to Overcome Insulin Resistance (IR) to live better & have an Energetic Life

Table of Contents

Introduction

I want to start by saying thank you and congratulations for purchasing the book, "The Insulin Resistance Diet: The Ultimate Guide to Overcome Insulin Resistance (IR) to live better & have an Energetic Life."

In this book, you will find information on what insulin resistance is- as well as the signs/symptoms used to diagnose this condition, and the various types of insulin resistance. You will also find proven strategies on how to obtain and maintain better health, even with the difficulties this condition can bring about.

When you have been diagnosed with an insulin resistance problem, you may feel confused and overwhelmed at first. However, once you realize that all you need to do in order to effectively manage your condition is to make some simple and healthy changes in your diet- you will emerge victorious in your battle against insulin resistance. The book you hold in your hands will guide you through understanding your situation. In addition, you will find a list of foods that are safe for you and a list of things that you should avoid.

So, what are you waiting for? Start reading and be sure to take notes- this book will definitely be the key to making your life so much sweeter.

Thanks again for purchasing this book, I hope you are able to get the information you need!

Insulin Resistance Explained

The condition of insulin resistance occurs when there is a decrease in the ability of the cells in your body to properly respond to insulin. This condition is the beginning of the body being unable to deal well with sugar- keep in mind that all carbs break down into sugar during the digestion process. One of the primary jobs of insulin in our bodies is to get cells to "open up" and take in glucose to store it as fat. However, in the condition of insulin resistance, when insulin comes knocking at the cell's doors, they don't "open up" and accept the glucose.

When this occurs, your body begins to put out more insulin in order to stabilize glucose levels in your blood so that the cells can use the glucose. Over a period of time, this leads to a condition referred to as "hyperinsulinemia"- which means that there is too much insulin in your blood. This leads to other issues, including making it much harder for your body to use stored fat for energy.

Causes of Insulin Resistance

We don't quite know the whole story, but we do know that genes do play a big role in this condition. In addition, two of the major contributors to the condition of insulin resistance are excess weight and lack of physical activity.

There are some experts that claim obesity, especially around the mid-section is one of the primary factors in causing insulin resistance. In the past, scientists believed that fat tissue served as energy storage, but more recent studies have revealed that belly fat actually produces hormones and other substances that can result in major health problems such as insulin resistance, cardiovascular disease, imbalanced cholesterol, and high blood pressure.

After all, the truth is that belly fat plays a major role in causing long-lasting (chronic) inflammation in your body. Over time, this can result in damage to your body- without any indication that there is a problem. Scientists have discovered that complicated interactions in your fat tissue will draw the immune cells to that area, which triggers inflammation. This inflammation, in turn, will contribute to the development of the condition of insulin resistance, cardiovascular disease, and type 2 diabetes. However, there is good news, studies have also proven that losing a few pounds can decrease insulin resistance and at least delay- if not prevent- the development of type 2 diabetes.

Some experts have found that physical activity is also involved in the condition of insulin resistance leading to type 2 diabetes. In your body, your muscles use more glucose than the rest of your tissues. When you're active, your muscles will burn the stored glucose and then fill the reserves will glucose pulled from your bloodstream, which keeps your blood sugar in balance.

Studies have proven that following a workout, your muscles will be much more sensitive to insulin, which reverses the insulin resistance and lowers your blood sugar levels. In addition, exercise can help your muscles to absorb more glucose without requiring the use of insulin. The more muscle you have, the more glucose you will be able to burn and keep blood sugar levels normalized.

Studies have also revealed that sleep problems- such as sleep apnea- when left untreated, can increase your risk of becoming obese. This means that you are at an increased risk of developing insulin resistance and type 2 diabetes. Individuals who work night shifts could be at a greater risk for developing these problems. Sleep apnea is a very common disorder. If you have sleep apnea, your breathing is interrupted while you sleep. You will most likely move out of a deep sleep and into a light sleep when your breathing becomes shallow or stops. This means that you will have poor sleep quality, which leads to excessive tiredness during the day.

Some of the other possible causes of insulin resistance are ethnicity, use of steroids, smoking cigarettes, age, some medications, and hormones.

Problems Caused by Insulin Resistance

The condition of insulin resistance is associated with the following conditions:

1) *You have excess belly fat.*

One of the most common signs that you have insulin resistance is weight gain around your middle section. Some individuals have an inherent apple shape; wherein they have lean and sculpted legs and arms as well as a full belly. Others observe that they gain weight around their middle section, which is absent during their younger years, once they hit middle age.

Know that your hips should be larger compared to your waist. If you are female, your waist measurement should not go beyond 75 percent of the size of your hips. Meanwhile, if you are male, your waist measurement should not go beyond 90 percent of the size of your hips.

If you are a man whose waist measures 36 inches, and no area of your lower body has a measurement of 40 inches, then you are likely to have a problem with insulin resistance.

On the other hand, if you are considered overweight, but your waist size is average when compared to your hip size, it is likely that your excess weight is well-distributed as well as balanced with muscle, reducing your chances of suffering from insulin resistance or eventually having a diabetic condition.

2) *Your health begins to decline.*

Insulin resistance can manifest itself in any of the following health issues:

- *Frequent infections*: May be an indicator and cause of insulin resistance.

- *Skin changes*: Certain changes in your skin texture or appearance, such as darkened areas in your skin folds and excessive skin tags, are indications of an insulin resistance problem.

- *Cataracts*: Patients suffering from both diabetes (type 1) and diabetes (type 2) increase their chances of developing cataracts. Individuals with insulin resistance could develop cataracts before the age of 70.

- *Reproductive problems*: Women who may not be overweight but have problems with their menstruation cycle and reproductive system (like poly cystic ovarian syndrome, or PCOS) can also be suffering from insulin resistance. If a woman was diagnosed with gestational diabetes while pregnant or gave birth to a baby weighing 9 pounds are more, she has a higher risk of developing insulin resistance.

- *Fatty liver*: In the past, a fatty liver was linked to issues with alcoholism, but in recent years, has been found in teens and even children and is an indicator of insulin resistance. The good news is that while a fatty liver due to alcoholism is usually a progressive condition, a fatty liver due to insulin resistance can be reversed with the help of the insulin resistance diet.

- *High blood pressure*: High blood pressure, along with fluid retention, is associated with insulin resistance, a result of elevated amounts of aldosterone in the body.

3) Lack of energy.

The most common sign of too much insulin in the body, which can lead to the condition of insulin resistance, is a problem with your blood sugar. You may be experiencing the phenomenon known as "sugar blues" when you feel either extremely excited or agitated after having eaten a sugary treat, or when you feel hungry again or sleepy after a meal.

After consuming a high-carb meal, your blood sugar spikes, which causes your body to produce more insulin- which then causes your blood sugar to drop quickly. This is what causes that sleepiness or lack of energy. When this cycle repeatedly occurs, you are at risk for developing insulin resistance.

The insulin resistance diet helps you address these issues and make it easier for you to lose your belly fat effectively, improve your health, and increase your energy levels. In the next chapter, you will find more information on the insulin resistance diet.

These conditions are all part of a culmination of problems associated with metabolic syndrome, or insulin resistance syndrome. Since these symptoms typically occur together, it's unclear as to what causes what, metabolic syndrome definitely puts you at a greater risk for developing heart disease and Type 2 diabetes.

Commonality of Insulin Resistance

This condition is much more common than you would probably think and is even becoming more so. In addition, the risk for developing this condition increases as you get older, which means that it could be related to the weight gain that commonly occurs during middle age.

One study did reveal that around 10 percent of the young adult population fits the criteria for being diagnosed with full metabolic syndrome. However, this figure rises to around 44 percent for those over the age of 60. Of course, it is much more likely that the condition of insulin resistance will occur without full-blown metabolic syndrome.

How to Know You Are Insulin Resistant

If you are overweight or obese, your risk for developing this condition increases, especially if this weight is carried in your abdominal region. In addition, if you have any of the signs and symptoms of metabolic syndrome as listed above, you are much more likely to develop insulin resistance. In addition, those who have a positive response to a diet that is reduced in carbohydrates is much more likely to be diagnosed as insulin resistant. Individuals who are diagnosed as insulin resistant should try reducing the carbs in their diet to get it under control. In order to help diagnose hyperinsulinemia and insulin resistant, medical experts often use a fasting insulin test.

What is Next?

When your pancreas is constantly having to pump out high levels of insulin, there will come a time when it can no longer do it. The common explanation of this is that the beta cells in your pancreas become "exhausted." However, it could be that the high levels of insulin and high levels of glucose in the blood have a damaging effect on the beta cells. Either way, at this time, your glucose levels will begin to rise more and more-which means that you are well on your way to developing Type 2 diabetes.

When your fasting blood sugar reaches 100 mg/dl, this is considered "prediabetes" and when it is 126 mg/dl, this is considered diabetes. As you can see, these are invisible lines on the road of an increasing inability for your body to be able to deal with sugar. First of all, insulin will become less and less effective- which means that there won't be enough insulin in your body to regulate the glucose. The sooner intervention occurs, the better off you will be.

Prediabetes and Type 2 Diabetes Defined

As mentioned in the previous chapter, the condition of insulin resistance can lead to prediabetes or type 2 diabetes. Following, you will find more information on those two conditions.

Prediabetes

The condition of prediabetes occurs when your blood sugar levels are higher than are considered normal, but not quite high enough to be diagnosed as type 2 diabetes. If you do not intervene and treat the condition, it is likely to develop into type 2 diabetes in 10 years or less. If you do have prediabetes, chances are that the long-term damage- especially to your circulatory system and your heart- have already begun.

However, have no fear- there really is good news. Prediabetes can be a wakeup call to get you to improve your overall health. Just because you have prediabetes does not mean that you will develop type 2 diabetes. By making some simple, healthy changes in your lifestyle such as: consuming a healthy diet, beginning an exercise program, and making sure that you maintain a healthy weight- you could be able to normalize your blood sugar levels.

Unfortunately, in most cases, there are no signs and symptoms for prediabetes. Of course, there are some signs that you could be at risk of developing type 2 diabetes such as a condition known as acanthosis nigricans, which refers to darkened skin on areas such as your armpits, elbows, knees, knuckles, and neck. There are some other signs and symptoms of type 2 diabetes that will be mentioned in the section on type 2 diabetes.

If you are concerned about diabetes or if you observe any signs/symptoms of type 2 diabetes as mentioned above, it's a good idea to make an appointment to see your physician. If you have any risk factors for prediabetes such as the following, you should ask your physician about blood glucose screening.

1) You are overweight and your BMI is over 25
2) You are not active
3) You are 45 or older
4) You have a family history of type 2 diabetes
5) You are a Pacific Islander, Hispanic, African-American, Asian-American, or American Indian
6) You were diagnosed with gestational diabetes while pregnant or your baby weighed 9 pounds or more
7) You have PCOS, or polycystic ovarian syndrome- which is a condition characterized by obesity, irregular periods, or excess hair growth
8) You have high blood pressure
9) Your HDL cholesterol is below 35 mg/dL or your triglycerides are over 250 mg/dL

The medical community is unsure of the exact cause of prediabetes, but it does seem that family history and genetics do play a critical role. Researchers have isolated some genes that do seem to be related to the condition of insulin resistance. As mentioned earlier, it seems that inactivity and abdominal fat are key factors in the development of prediabetes.

While the cause may not be clear, what is clear is that individuals who have the condition of prediabetes are unable to process glucose properly. This means that the sugar builds up in their blood instead of doing its job of fueling cells in the muscles and other tissues. Keep in mind that most of the glucose in your body does come from the foods you are eating- which means that its best if you consume a healthy diet- specifically carbs. All foods that contain carbs can have an effect on your blood sugar levels- it doesn't have to be sweet.

During the process of digestion, the sugar will enter your bloodstream. Your pancreas produces insulin- which then helps the sugar to get into the cells of your muscles and tissues, which means it can be used for energy. This means that insulin decreases the levels of sugar in your blood. As the sugar levels drop, the secretion of insulin by your pancreas will as well.

However, in the condition of prediabetes, this process begins to malfunction. The sugar, instead of fueling cells in your muscles and tissues, begins to build up in your blood. This is either because your pancreas isn't making enough insulin, your cells have become resistant to insulin, or a combination of both.

A progression to type 2 diabetes is a very serious consequence that comes when you don't make sure to treat your prediabetes. The condition of type 2 diabetes can lead to more serious health complications as mentioned in Chapter 1.

1) High cholesterol
2) High blood pressure
3) Heart disease
4) Kidney disease
5) Stroke
6) Amputations
7) Blindness

If you believe you may be at risk for developing prediabetes, chances are you will start by seeing your general practitioner. He or she may then refer you to an endocrinologist, who specializes in diabetic conditions.

When you go see your physician, you will most likely be asked a few questions, such as the following:

1) Have you noticed a recent change in your weight?
2) Do you get exercise on a regular basis? If you do: how often and for how long?
3) Do you know if you have a family history of diabetes or diabetic conditions?

Following are a few suggestions to help you get ready for your doctor visit.

1) Make sure that you know about any pre-appointment restrictions: when you make your appointment, make sure to ask if there's anything you need to or can do in advance, such as put some restrictions on your diet. Chances are that you will be asked to fast for at least eight hours before so that the physician can measure your fasting blood sugar.
2) Be sure to write down any symptoms you are having, including those that seem to be unrelated to the reason you made the appointment.
3) Bring a list of your medications, including any OTC vitamins/supplements.
4) If you have any questions for your physician, be sure to bring a list of those too. Here are some that you might want to consider:
   a. Is there something I can do to prevent prediabetes from developing into type 2 diabetes?
   b. Is there any medications I can take to control it?
   c. What side effects can I expect from the medications?
   d. What is the best way to manage all of my conditions together?
   e. How much exercise should I be getting on a daily/weekly basis?
   f. Is there any food/foods I should be avoiding? Will I still be able to eat sugary snacks?
   g. Will I need to get in touch with a dietician?
   h. Do you have any printed materials I can take with me or perhaps direct me to a website for more information?

Of course, if you have other questions besides these, don't feel bad about asking them. In addition, make sure that you understand your physician's answers before you leave.

Type 2 Diabetes

Once referred to as adult-onset diabetes or noninsulin dependent diabetes, the condition of type 2 diabetes is a chronic one that has an effect on the way your body processes sugar- which is an important source of fuel for your body's cells.

In the condition of type 2 diabetes, your body is either resistant to the effects of insulin or your pancreas is not producing enough insulin to regulate blood sugar levels.

While the condition of type 2 diabetes is much more common in adults, it is increasingly affecting children as the epidemic of childhood obesity is ever increasing. There is no cure for this condition, but you can manage it by simply eating well, getting adequate exercise, and making sure that you maintain a healthy weight for your age and frame. However, if diet and exercise are not enough to keep your blood sugar regulated, your physician may recommend insulin therapy or diabetes medications.

As mentioned earlier, there are some signs and symptoms that you have type 2 diabetes. Keep in mind that these typically develop slowly. The truth is that you may have this condition for several years before you even realize it. Here are some of the signs and symptoms of the condition of type 2 diabetes:

1) An increase in thirst and urination: when sugar starts building up in your bloodstream, this results in fluid being pulled from your tissues. This will leave you feeling extra thirsty- which means you will be drinking and urinating much more often than usual.
2) An increase in hunger: when your body is not providing enough insulin to move the sugar into your cells, muscles and organs will become depleted of energy- which leads to intense hunger.
3) An increase in weight loss: even though you're eating more because you're so hungry, you're still losing

weight. Since your body is not metabolizing glucose properly to fuel it, you are burning alternative fuels that are stored in muscles and fat. As the excess glucose is released in your urine, you are also losing calories.

4) An increase in fatigue: when your cells are not getting the sugar they need for energy, you begin to feel more tired and irritable than usual.

5) Blurry vision: when your blood sugar begins to rise and becomes too high, your body starts pulling fluid from various areas, which can include the lenses of your eyes, which has an effect on your ability to focus.

6) Areas of darkened skin: as mentioned earlier, in some cases, individuals with the condition of type 2 diabetes have patches of darkened skin in the folds/creases of their bodies. This is a condition known as acanthosis nigricans and could be a sign that your body is insulin resistant.

The condition of type 2 diabetes develops when your body becomes resistant to insulin or your pancreas ceases producing enough. Again, it's not really clear on why this occurs, but it does seem that genetic and environmental factors seem to contribute.

The very same factors increase your risk of developing prediabetes and type 2 diabetes. These include:

1) Weight: being overweight/obese is one of the primary risk factors for diabetic conditions. The more fatty tissue you have, the more likely your cells are to become resistant to insulin.

2) Waist Size: having a large waist size can be indicative of insulin resistance. This risk increases in men who have a waist size larger than 40 inches and for women with a waist size larger than 35.

3) Physical Inactivity: the less physically active you are, the more likely you are to develop diabetic conditions. Physical activity is great for controlling your weight, using up glucose as

energy, and actually makes your cells more sensitive to the effects of insulin.

4) Age: while it's true that diabetic conditions can develop at any age, the risk for prediabetes or type 2 diabetes increases as you get older-especially after the age of 45. This is likely due to the fact that older individuals tend to exercise less, which means they gain weight and lose muscle mass.

5) Family History: if you have a parent or sibling with type 2 diabetes, your risk for developing prediabetes and type 2 diabetes increases.

6) Race: while there doesn't seem to be a clear reason why, some races seem to have a greater likelihood of developing diabetic conditions.

7) Gestational Diabetes: if you were diagnosed with gestational diabetes when you were pregnant, your risk of later developing diabetic conditions increases. If your baby weighed more than 9 pounds, you're also at an increased risk of developing a diabetic condition.

8) PCOS: women who have been diagnosed with PCOS, or polycystic ovarian syndrome, are at a greater risk for developing diabetic conditions.

9) Poor Sleep: researchers have found that sleep problems increase an individual's risk of developing diabetic conditions. This includes those who work changing shifts or night shifts.

Best Foods to Choose for Insulin Resistance

When you have been diagnosed with the condition of insulin resistance, you must always keep in mind that in addition to how much you are eating- the way you are eating also has a major impact on your weight. There are certain foods that can help you to get fit and keep your glucose levels under control- which could possibly help you to avoid diabetic conditions. Following are just a few of the foods which you can mix and match to create solid, fulfilling meals.

Vegetables

Veggies are low in calories and starches- this means they are the perfect form of nourishment for those who are trying to gain/maintain control of their blood glucose levels. The best choice are solid veggies because veggie juices- while they may seem like a good idea- are not going to fill you up as quickly as fresh, crisp veggies. Some great options are tomatoes, spinach, yams, collard greens, corn, and even kale.

Fruits

If you want to make sure you're getting an adequate amount of fiber, vitamins, and minerals, crunch on some fruits. While it's best to choose fresh, you can choose canned- as long as there is no added sugar. Organic fruits are best because they will gradually increase your blood glucose levels. Some popular options are apples, bananas, grapes, plums, and peaches. However, you must keep in mind that it's best to avoid natural fruit juices because they can cause your glucose levels to spike- which is what you don't want to happen.

Dairy

Dairy is great for providing you with the calcium you need to make sure that your teeth and bones stay healthy. However, it's best to choose dairy products that are fat-free or low-fat. This is because insulin resistance tends to compound when you consume full-fat dairy products. If you are lactose intolerant, you may want to choose products such as sustained soy milk, rice milk, or almond milk.

Whole Grains

Whole grains are packed with fiber, vitamins, and minerals. This means they are perfect for controlling diabetic conditions. In order to ensure that you're getting the right amount of what you need, you must choose items such as whole wheat flour, whole oats, bulgar, whole grain corn, and chestnut rice. In addition, you can also choose products containing whole grains, whole rye, wild rice, quinoa, and herbs.

Nuts

Nuts, seeds, and nut/seed margarines give you plenty of solids, magnesium, protein, and fiber. In addition, nuts/seeds are low in starches, which is an advantage if you are attempting to control your blood glucose levels. There are a few nuts/seeds such as walnuts and flax seeds that also contain heart-healthy omega-3 unsaturated fats. Still, while a good choice, you must be mindful of the amount of nuts/seeds you consume because nuts are very high in calories- which can lead to weight gain. Also, you want to make sure you're aware of how the nuts/seeds are prepared. There are a few nut/seed snacks and spreads out there that also contain high levels of sugar and sodium- which means they're not as healthy.

Beans

Beans are full of fiber and are excellent choices because they raise glucose levels gradually- which makes them good for those who are dealing with the condition of insulin resistance. Some great options are pinto, lima, and dark beans. If you don't have a whole lot of time to prepare, canned beans are a decent option to dried beans. However, you must make sure that you drain and flush them because they can contain high levels of sodium.

Fish

A common condition of those with diabetes are coronary problems. Fish are full of omega-3 unsaturated fats and can decrease your risk for developing these problems. Fish rich in omega-3 include salmon, mackerel, saltwater fish, sardines, arc trout, tilapia, cod, wallow, halibut, and haddock are all excellent choices. If you prefer shellfish, you can try lobster, scallops, shrimp, shellfish, mollusks, or crabs, However, you must also keep in mind that these foods also are typically high in cholesterol. In addition, as with any other foods, you want to avoid fish that is broiled or breaded.

Poultry

In order to make sure your poultry is clean, peel and throw out the skin. The skin of poultry has more fat than the meat does. Choose chicken breasts, turkey, or Cornish hen. When you eat eggs, choose egg whites, as they are much lower in calories than the whole egg- and they don't contain fat.

Other Lean Meats

Even if you do have insulin resistance, you can still eat other lean meats such as pork, veal, sheep, and hamburger. Great choices are pork tenderloins, veal loin, sheep legs, or a hamburger with the fat trimmed.

Planning your insulin resistance diet-friendly meals on a daily basis can be very challenging. Here are some menu ideas to help you be successful:

Meal Ideas for an Insulin Resistance Diet

While it's always a good idea to pay attention to what you're eating- when you've been diagnosed with insulin resistance, it's even more critical. In the previous chapters, you learned about what insulin resistance is, what prediabetes and type 2 diabetes are, and the best foods to choose for an insulin resistance diet. In this chapter, you will find some great meal ideas for your insulin resistance diet. This will help you start putting some of this into action in your life and to get your condition under control.

Breakfast Ideas

You've always heard that breakfast is the most important meal of the day. That same saying holds true for those who are insulin resistant. You want to start your day with something that is going to sustain you through the morning and get you to your lunch time. Here are some ideas:

1. Eggs

Eggs have been very common breakfast items for a variety of reasons: they're inexpensive, they're easy to cook, they can be prepared in a variety of ways, and they are low in calories and full of nutrients.

2. Bacon

While bacon is full of fat, it is allowed in the insulin resistance diet. Combine bacon bits with some cheese, mushrooms, bell peppers, or scallions in a breakfast omelet.

3. Cereals

When you buy cereals, choose hypoglycemic index options. These include muesli, granola, oatmeal (coarsely flaked), or all-bran variants, which will not cause your blood sugar levels to shoot up.

4. Coffee

Thankfully, you're not going to have to give up your morning coffee when you go on the insulin resistance diet. While it's true that green tea tastes great in the morning as well, and the benefits that it can provide are numerous and well-documented, nothing beats having good old coffee to start your day. If you feel it would help you better control your insulin resistance problems, you can try decaffeinated coffee. However, you must keep in mind that you don't need to add sugar to your coffee. Instead, try stevia or other natural sugar substitutes. If you have to use creamer in your coffee, choose cream or milk over artificial creamers.

Lunch Ideas

Lunch is your mid-day meal. This is what you need to sustain you for the rest of the day. As with every other meal, you want to make sure you're choosing foods that are safe for individuals with insulin resistance. Following are some great ideas for lunch. Some of them require a decent amount of time and others you can just throw together before heading out the door to work.

1. Sandwich

Sandwiches are great options for lunch- but only if you eat just one. Choose high-fiber, low glycemic index breads such as rye or sourdough. In addition, make sure that the filling is a lean protein.

2. Salad

You can make a salad for a delicious lunch, especially if you have plenty of time in the morning. Include chicken pieces, lean ham cuts, turkey slices, roast beef bits, cheese cubes, and/or tuna chunks in the mix. Then add in tomatoes, lettuce, avocado slices, pine nuts, cilantro/coriander sprigs, or mixed beans. If you use the beans, be sure to rinse them first to get rid of the extra starch.

3. Salad dressing

Salads always taste better with dressing, but you do have to pay attention to the label on your dressings. Be sure to pay attention to the sugar and carbohydrates in the dressing so that you can avoid choices that are high in carbohydrates. Instead, choose low-carb options such as Caesar, vinaigrettes, or balsamic dressings. While it's true that these are higher in fat, your primary concern is the carbohydrates, since you're on an insulin resistance diet.

4. Soup

Especially on a cold day, warm soup is satisfyingly delicious. When you are on the insulin resistance diet, try making a homemade soup so that you can be sure about everything that goes into it. For the base, choose non-starchy veggies and lean proteins. If you like a thick soup, there are other options besides potatoes, such as beans, quinoa, barley, chickpeas, and lentils to achieve the same results.

Snack Ideas

When you still have a bit of time between lunch and dinner, but you're starting to get a bit hungry, you do have options. This way, you won't be starving when dinnertime comes around and end up eating too much- or not the right things for you.

1. Almonds

On the insulin resistance diet, you can eat almonds- but you have to do so in moderation. You must limit yourself to about ten pieces though- or try other nuts, but also practice moderation with them as well.

2. Cheese

Cheese is always an excellent choice for a snack. After all, it tastes great and it keeps you from experiencing food cravings between meals. A few spoonfuls of cottage cheese eaten on its own or some shredded Parmesan eaten with a celery stick- say no to crackers- will always be better than a chocolate chip cookie.

3. Peanut butter

Even with the high amount of fat (and calories) it contains, peanut butter can still be part of your insulin resistance diet. You can eat it by the spoonful (one or two), and add a little extra flavor by adding a little salt.

Dinner Ideas

Finally, comes dinner time. This is your last meal of the day- make it a good one, but not too heavy. You want to be full and to make sure you can sustain your blood sugar through the night, but you don't want to overeat or eat something that will cause your blood sugar level to crash.

1. Vegetables

Cauliflower is a great veggie base for your meals. Cook until tender and mash with a fork. Any leftovers can be used to create a yummy cauliflower cheese bake the following day. In addition to cauliflower, you can use alfalfa, eggplant, pumpkin, zucchini, button squash, spaghetti squash, bean sprouts, red peppers, and onions. These can all be seasoned with garlic, lemon juice, and herbs.

2. Coconut soup

Spice up your insulin resistance diet menu with chicken cooked in coconut soup. However, keep in mind that you must only eat one bowl of this yummy soup.

3. Slow cooker meals

When you go on an insulin resistance diet, a slow cooker is a great thing to have- especially if you don't have a whole lot of time to cook at the end of your day. Simply chop up your vegetables and meat in the morning, place them in the slow cooker before heading to work, and come home to a delicious meal at dinner time. However, when creating your slow cooker meals, leave out the potatoes, instead choosing beans or other non-starchy veggies. Remember to always toss in some protein into your mix too.

4. Barbecue

If you prefer, you can always eat a huge serving of yummy salad and barbequed fish, prawns, or lean meats.

Other Food Ideas

If you find that none of the above really sounds appealing to you, there are a few other options as well. Following are a few common foods/spices that you can use to supplement your insulin resistance diet.

1. Blueberries

Insulin levels- and belly fat- can be reduced by as much as 22 percent by enjoying a really delicious blueberry smoothie. One study revealed that blueberries are rich in bioactive substances that, when consumed on a daily basis, can increase your insulin sensitivity, which decreases your risk of developing diabetes. In addition, researchers observed that individuals who are obese, but not diagnosed as diabetic, also benefit from a 22 percent reduction in insulin resistance when they drank a blueberry smoothie every day for six weeks.

2. Cinnamon

By adding just a teaspoonful of cinnamon to your diet on a daily basis for a period of twenty days, you can decrease your insulin resistance. You can easily do this by infusing your blueberry smoothies with one to six grams of cinnamon on a daily basis for 40 days. This will also reduce your blood sugar levels by as much as 20 percent. Research has proven that cinnamon not only reduces blood sugar levels, but also LDL cholesterol and total cholesterol levels in those who are suffering from type 2 diabetes.

3. Tart cherries

If you snack on tart cherries for a period of three months, you'll see a reduction in your insulin resistance. Research done on rats has shown that tart cherries not only reduce insulin resistance, but also reduce belly fat and improve overall health. You can get these benefits whether you eat them alone or adding one serving of them to your smoothies, ½ cup with a bit of Greek yogurt, or eating 1 tablespoon of mixed nuts combined with ¼ cup of tart cherries.

Things to Keep in Mind about the Insulin Resistance Diet

When you have been diagnosed with the condition of insulin resistance and you are required to go on the insulin resistance diet, you may be afraid that your food choices will become limited- which will have a major effect on your energy levels. There is a bit of truth to this thought- especially since your body is going to need to adjust to the changes you are going to be applying in your diet. However, there are some things you can do to ease your way into this new way of life without too much of a hassle.

Diet Tips

The following tips help you address sugar cravings as well as help you prevent any sudden drops in your energy levels.

1. Deal with your sugar cravings wisely.

Having those cravings for sugar and other sweets is usually a sign that your body is not receiving the proper balance of proteins and carbohydrates. Many people frequently experience the need to snack by mid-afternoon, but having extreme cravings for sugar is not normal and usually indicates that your body is missing out on something from your diet. If you feel that sugar cravings can hit you whenever afternoon rolls around, consider adding more fish, low-fat dairy, or lean meat to your lunch fare.

2. Have some green tea.

Some individuals have found drinking green tea to be an effective way for them to curb their sugar cravings.

3. Fish oil helps.

Fish oil allows your cells to respond in a more efficient manner to your digestive hormones, and this results in your body requiring less insulin.

4. Don't forget to take your vitamin D.

Taking vitamin D (4000 IU) may help you reduce your insulin resistance problem in 6 months, as indicated in a published study done on women. The same women improved their insulin sensitivity issues after taking vitamin D supplements over a period of 6 months.

5. Always take your zinc.

You may be able to improve your insulin levels in eight days if you simply take your zinc every day. This mineral plays a major role in the functioning of as many as 200 enzymes in your body, which is why zinc deficiency is no laughing matter. The recommended daily dosage for zinc supplements is 15 to 25 milligrams.

6. Don't eliminate fat.

Trying to skimp on your fat intake will not get you anywhere, particularly when the insulin resistance diet is concerned. Your body needs fat to digest your food and absorb the nutrients it provides. Consuming fats along with protein also helps improve your gut motility, especially when you combine it with some thorough chewing of your food as well as a post-eating walk.

7. Take advantage of salt.

Salt plays a significant role in keeping your bowel movement regular. You can get adequate salt from your main dishes, homemade broths, and 200 to 800-milligram magnesium supplements (if you have constipation problems).

8. Go for probiotic foods.

Incorporating probiotic foods in your insulin resistance diet is an effective way of carefully introducing enzymes needed by your digestive system. Including sauerkraut in your daily menu is just one of the easiest things you can do to achieve that.

9. Feed your brain with L-glutamine.

Being on the insulin resistance diet can make you feel groggy at times, especially in the early stages. Combat the grogginess with a daily supplement of L-glutamine (at a dosage of 500 to 10,000 milligrams). You also benefit from the ability of L-glutamine to maintain gut health, which you need while adapting to the insulin resistance diet.

10. Drink plenty of water.

Adequate water helps your body carry out its numerous functions effectively and efficiently, which in turn helps it produce more energy. Drinking enough water also ensures that you avoid getting headaches and migraines, which can definitely drain you of your energy. Water as a beverage also helps you control your sugar cravings, letting you avoid the dreaded slump after a sudden sugar high. Lastly, drinking enough water prevents your body from suffering from dehydration (especially during and after exercise), which leads to fatigue.

Breaking Down the Insulin Resistance Diet

When it comes to the insulin resistance diet, here are some things that you need to know to help you be able to stay on track. Following, you will find a breakdown of the insulin resistance diet- and perhaps be able to understand it and follow it a little bit better.

1. Whenever you are hungry, eat meat.

Unprocessed meats: You can take your pick from the following: ham, lamb, pork, bacon, beef, venison, veal, and elk.

Processed meats: Checking labels is important in choosing processed meats. Keep in mind that you should aim to keep your carb count at only one gram in one serving. If your budget allows, know that it is best to go for grass-fed processed meats instead of those that are grain-finished. You should also try enjoying the fat that is on your meats since it helps your digestive process, allows your body to absorb nutrients better, and improves your overall health.

Eggs: You are better off eating whole eggs that are produced by pasture-raised chickens.

Poultry: Your poultry choices include turkey, chicken, duck, and other fowl.

Fish and shellfish: Wild salmon and tuna are just some of the seafood choices you can incorporate in your insulin resistance diet.

2. Don't exclude fat from your meals.

Healthy fats: Organic butter, organic lard, and all other healthful types of oils (These should be cold-pressed; avoid the hydrogenated ones like margarine.) and fats are allowed in the insulin resistance diet.

Frying oils: When cooking fried dishes, use healthy fats like coconut oil, ghee, lard, and other oils that remain solid at room temperature.

Salad dressings: Your salad dressings are best made with lemon juice, vinegar, or olive oil. They are healthier options compared to prepared dressings (even if they may be labeled "light") that are not only typically made using oils that are genetically modified, but also contain plenty of carbs.

3. Include these foods in your daily diet:

Vegetables: Aim to eat one cup (uncooked measurement) of zucchini, tomatoes, bean sprouts, Brussels sprouts, eggplant, asparagus, rhubarb, sugar snap peas, celery, artichokes, pumpkin, okra, shallots, summer squash, broccoli, cauliflower, cucumber, onions, snow peas, green beans, leeks, peppers, wax beans, jicama, or mushrooms.

Greens: Eat a daily serving of two cups (measured raw) of cooked or raw green leafy vegetables. You will be able to benefit the most from greens if you eat them with some kind of fat, such as melted grass-fed butter.

Homemade broth soup: You need to replenish your body's lost minerals on a daily basis, and soup helps you achieve this. Opt for homemade broth as this lets you control the amount of salt you put in to suit your taste as well as avoid going overboard.

4. Go easy on these foods allowed in your diet:

Butter and cream (organic): Know that the insulin resistance diet does allow you to enjoy consuming butter and cream (whipping cream, not half-and-half). Just remember that you are limited by the premise that you have to eat them only after you have had your fill of the other healthy food choices listed above.

Cheese (organic): If you are a cheese lover, you will love the fact that the insulin resistance diet allows you to have a daily serving of four ounces of organic cheese. Stay away from the processed ones.

Snacks: If you absolutely cannot do without deli meats, know that you can still eat (in limited portions) pepperoni and sausage. You can also snack on delicious deviled eggs.

Avocado: The insulin resistance diet allows you to enjoy eating half of an avocado on a daily basis.

Lime juice/lemon juice: Include up to about four teaspoons of lime juice or lemon juice in your daily dishes or beverages.

Pickles: Dill pickles that are made without any added sugar can be included in your insulin resistance diet, at about one to two servings daily.

Mayonnaise: Under the insulin resistance diet, you are allowed to have about one to four tablespoons of mayonnaise per day.

Olives: Have your fill of olives – as much as six green or black ones per day.

Tamari: Tamari is also allowed – you can consume as much as four tablespoons daily.

5. Do away with these foods:

Starches: Starches not allowed under the insulin resistance diet include cereals, breads, grains, flour, pasta, rice, cornstarch, bagels, beans (black, Lima, Pinto, and other slow-cooked varieties) and other starchy vegetables, peas, root vegetables, and potatoes (as well as all kinds of potato products).

Sugars (in all forms): In the insulin resistance diet, this covers both the simple and complex carbohydrates. Include in your diet fiber-rich and nutritionally-dense vegetables, and avoid at all costs maple syrup, corn syrup, fruit as well as fruit juices, milk, honey, molasses, table sugar, flavored yogurts, and beer.

Inflammatory oils: Inflammatory oils, which include canola oil, cottonseed oil, and soybean oil, contribute to your difficulty in losing belly fat as well as increase your risk of having cancer and suffering from a degenerative disease.

Menu for the Insulin Resistance Diet

Your hormones determine the amount of fat your body stores as well as where your body stores it. If you are suffering from mild to serious health issues due to being overweight or obese, it's quite possible that high insulin levels are somehow involved. In order to efficiently drop your insulin levels, as well as improve your overall health, consider the following food/recipe ideas.

BREAKFAST

Basturma Egg Cups

Ingredients:

- 2 eggs
- 5 thin slices of basturma

Instructions:

Preheat your pan about to 320 degrees Fahrenheit. Then using 2 basturma cuts, line silicone muffin mold to form a cross pattern. Next, gently break the egg into a bowl and cut the remaining slice of basturma into small pieces and put in the bowl with the egg. Whisk the egg with the bits of basturma then gently pour into muffin pan. Bake it for approximately 10-15 minutes depending upon how you like your eggs. And lastly, present it with a serving of mixed greens.

Nutrition Facts:

Calories: 169
Total fat: 4g
Total carbs: 5g
Protein: 229g

The Big Breakfast Recipe

Ingredients:

- 2 cherry tomatoes
- A sprinkle of oregano
- 1 mushroom
- 10 pc baby spinach leaves
- 2 thin slices of ham
- 1 egg
- 1 slice of bread

Instructions:

Cut all the tomatoes in half and grill for 5 minutes. If you don't care for grilled veggies, you can bake them instead. In a pan, sauté mushrooms and add just a little water to ensure tenderness. Add spinach and stir. Let it boil for about 5 minutes. Set aside. Place your egg in a bag and place it in the water. Cook until done, according to your taste. While your egg is cooking, place bread in toaster. Place toast on plate, top with ham, egg, tomato, mushrooms, and spinach.

Nutrition Facts:

Calories: 367
Total fat: 9.6
Cholesterol: 222
Sodium: 769
Potassium: 25
Total carbs: 51.2
Sugars: 4.1
Protein: 7.9
Vitamin A: 8%
Calcium: 11%
Iron: 21%

Low-Sodium Breakfast Sausage

Ingredients:

- 8 ounces lean fresh ground pork
- 2 tablespoons chicken stock
- 1/2 teaspoon thyme, dried
- 1/4 teaspoon sage, dried
- 1/2 teaspoon black pepper
- 1/2 teaspoon red pepper flakes

Instructions:

In a large mixing bowl, combine all ingredients and mix thoroughly. While mixing, ingredients will start to form a ball. Create meatballs from the mixture and place them on a piece of wax paper- use the other side to flatten the balls. Once your patties are formed, you can place them in your preheated nonstick pan to fry them. Fry them on medium high heat for five minutes on each side. Before eating, make sure they are cooked thoroughly.

Nutrition Facts:

Calories: 147.7
Total fat: 11.1 g
Cholesterol: 37.5 mg
Sodium: 36 mg
Dietary fiber: .2 g
Protein: 10.1 g

Healthy Breakfast Cookie

Ingredients:

- 2 large eggs, beaten
- 1/2 cup of honey
- 1/4 cup of butter
- 1 cup grated carrots
- 1/2 cup raisins
- 1 cup walnuts, chopped
- 1/2 cup dried apricots, chopped
- 1 cup all-purpose flour
- 1 cup rolled oats
- 1 tsp Nutmeg
- 1 tsp Cinnamon

Instructions:

In a large mixing bowl, combine all the dry ingredients and mix well. Combine the raisins, walnuts and Apricots to the dried ingredients and gradually stir in your wet ingredients. Set mixture aside. Prepare your cookie sheet and form balls from the dough with a scooper. Place on cookie sheet and flatten slightly. Place in preheated oven and bake for 15 to 20 minutes.

Nutrition Facts:
Calories: 111.1
Total fat: 5 mg
Cholesterol: 18 mg
Sodium 39.9 mg
Total carbs: 16.2 g
Dietary fiber: 1.2 g
Protein: 2.1 g

Granola Breakfast Bars

Ingredients:

- 2 1/4 cups old fashioned oats
- 1/2 cup whole wheat flour
- 1/2 teaspoon baking soda
- 1/2 teaspoon vanilla
- 5 tablespoons applesauce
- 1/4 cup honey
- 1/4 cup brown sugar
- 1/2 cup additions
- chopped nuts

Instructions:

Preheat your oven to 350 degrees Fahrenheit. Combine all ingredients, making sure to completely incorporate them. Grease an 8x8 pan and pour in mixture. You can use a spatula to even it out. Bake for 15 to 20 minutes or until firm. The top should be golden and crispy. Cut into small bars before serving.

Nutrition Facts:
Calories: 137
Total fat: 1.1 g
Sodium: 110.2 mg
Total carbs: 31.2 g
Dietary fibers: 2.3 g
Protein: 10.1 g

Breakfast Smoothies

Ingredients:

- 1 Cup orange juice
- 1 Cup fresh berries
- 6-8 oz. plain yogurt
- 1 banana

Instructions:

Blend the juice with ice and gradually add in your yogurt on low. Add the fruits such as banana and berries. You'll get the best results with frozen fruits. You may use any other fruit combination to create a new flavored smoothie. Serve cold.

Nutrition Facts:

Calories: 196
Total fat: .6 g
Cholesterol: 2.5 mg
Sodium: 154.3 mg
Total carbs: 38.7 g
Dietary fiber: 4.1 g
Protein: 4.7 g

Turkey Bacon Breakfast Rolls

Ingredients:

- 1 tube whole wheat dough
- 3 slices cooked turkey bacon
- 1 teaspoon dried thyme

Instructions:

Preheat oven to 350 degrees Fahrenheit. Using a clean cutting/kneading board, dust on a handful of flour. Place dough on board and start kneading until it has spread out onto the surface of the board. Once ready, arrange bacon on it, then add thyme. Roll dough into a pinwheel and place on baking sheet. Be sure to spray your baking sheet with oil and dust it with flour to avoid sticking. Bake for 15 to 20 minutes, or until golden brown. Slice and serve.

Nutrition Facts:

Calories: 137.8
Total fat: 2.8 g
Cholesterol: 7.5 mg
Sodium: 390 mg
Total carbs: 24.1 g
Dietary fiber: 1 g
Protein: 5 g

Breakfast Muffin Bonanza

Ingredients:

- 1 cup packed brown sugar
- 1/2 cup canola or vegetable oil
- 1 cup low fat buttermilk
- 1 egg
- 2 tbsp. molasses
- 1-1/2 cups natural bran
- 2/3 cup flour
- 1/2 cup wheat germ
- 1/4 cup sesame seeds
- 1/4 cup flax seeds
- 1 tsp baking soda
- 1/2 tsp salt
- 1/2 tsp cinnamon
- 1 cup raisins

Instructions:

Preheat oven to 400 degrees Fahrenheit. In a large mixing bowl, combine dry ingredients, making sure they are sifted well. Add wet ingredients while mixing to ensure that all ingredients are well blended. Once batter is ready, you can grease you muffin tin and start spooning batter into them. Bake for 20 to 25 minutes, or until muffins start to rise. Depending on your mood, these are great hot or cold.

Nutrition Facts:

Calories: 308.8
Total fat: 13.4 g
Cholesterol: 16.4 mg
Sodium: 240.4 mg
Total carbs: 46.8 g
Dietary fiber: 6 g
Protein: 5.8

Bacon & Cheddar Breakfast Muffins

Ingredients:

- 1 cup whole wheat flour
- 1/3 cup rolled oats
- 1 Tbs. baking powder
- 1/2 Tsp. salt
- 6 jumbo eggs
- 1/4 cup apple sauce
- 1/2 cup cheddar cheese (shredded)
- 1/2 cup cooked chopped bacon
- 1/4 cup parsley
- 1/4 tsp Pepper
- 1/4 tsp ground cinnamon

Instructions:

Preheat oven to about 350 degrees Fahrenheit. In a large mixing bowl, using a spatula, combine all dry ingredients. Of course, if you have an electric mixer, you can use that instead. Add wet ingredients. When wet and dry are well mixed, you can add in the cheese, bacon, and parsley. Grease muffin pan before pouring batter. Bake for 20 to 25 minutes or until slightly browned. While still hot, remove from pan to avoid sticking. You can serve hot or cold.

Nutrition Facts:

Calories: 123.3
Total fat: 5 g
Cholesterol: 126 mg
Sodium: 295.1 mg
Total carbs: 9.9 g
Dietary fiber: 1.5 g
Protein: 6.9 g

Breakfast Casserole

Ingredients:

- 12 ounces breakfast sausage
- 1 teaspoon chicken broth
- 4 1/2 cups whole-wheat bread cubes
- 8 ounces low fat cheddar cheese
- 1 teaspoon mustard powder
- 2 large whole eggs
- 4 egg whites
- 2 cups low fat milk

Instructions:

Preheat oven to 350 degrees Fahrenheit. In a bowl, combine all eggs, egg whites, milk, and chicken broth. In a separate bowl, mix the bread cubes, sausage, cheese, and mustard. Season with salt if desired. Place bread/sausage mixture on a nonstick pan and drizzle wet ingredients on top. Bake for 30 to 45 minutes. Serve hot.

Nutrition Facts:

Calories: 308.3
Total fat: 12.4 g
Cholesterol: 84.9 mg
Sodium: 669.2 mg
Total carbs: 21.2 g
Dietary fiber: 2 g
Protein: 27.7 g

LUNCH

Simple Bento Lunch

Ingredients:

- 1c Rice cooked
- 10 blackberries
- 1c mixed green peas
- 6 turkey meatballs
- 1 soy sauce sachet

Instructions:

Prepare bento box, ensuring that it is clean and free of dirt. Wipe dry before proceeding to the next step. In a bowl, place your rice and allow to cool. Once rice is cool, start forming your rice balls. Arrange rice and meat balls according to taste and add veggies and berries on the side. You can place a soy sauce packet on the side just in case you want to add more flavor.

Nutrition Facts:
Calories: 432.6
Total fat: 10.5 g
Cholesterol: 50 mg
Sodium: 1 845.2 mg
Total carbs: 62 g
Dietary fiber: 11.6 g
Protein: 26.1

Hummus Pita

Ingredients:

- 2 Whole Wheat Pita
- 4 Tbsp. Hummus
- 1/4 Cup Shredded Carrots
- 4 slices of tomato
- 1 slice low Fat Pepper Cheese
- 1/2 Cup Sprouts

Instructions:

Combine all other ingredients except the pita bread in a bowl. Set into the bread and you may now roll or fold it. Should be eaten as soon as you can to prevent the pita bread from getting stale.

Nutrition Facts:
Calories: 282.1
Total fat: 12.4 g
Cholesterol: 10 mg
Sodium: 762.2 mg
Total carbs: 32.6 g
Dietary fibers: 12.2 g
Protein: 23.9 g

Easy Egg Recipe

Ingredients:
- 2 large eggs
- 1 large potatoes, peeled and cut into small cubes
- 1 large red tomato, sliced
- 1/2 cucumber, peeled and sliced

Instructions:

Rinse the potatoes under running water to remove the soil and dirt in it. Cut into cubes for fast cooking. In a pan cook the potatoes over a medium-high heat and wait until firm and tender. Pour in the beaten eggs to the potatoes like cooking an omelet. Serve with tomatoes and cucumber. This is optional.

Nutrition Facts:
Calories: 317
Total fat: 10.9 g
Cholesterol: 425 mg
Sodium: 153.8 mg
Total carbs: 38.4 g
Dietary fiber: 6.1 g
Protein: 17.8 g

Easy Lunch

Ingredients:

- Potato, Boiled 100 grams
- Tomato & Chili Sauce 50 grams
- Spinach 1 cup
- Onions, raw, .5 cup, chopped
- Swede, 1 serving
- mature cheese, 25 grams

Instructions:

Simply cook all in the usual way without adding oil and butter. Pile into boxes the top with the raw spinach. When reheating microwave for 4 min.

Nutrition Facts:
Calories: 34.6
Total fat; 12 g
Sodium: 59.8 mg
Total carbs: 28.7 g
Dietary fiber: 4.9 g
Protein: 29.4 g

Sausage and Vegetable Combination

Ingredients:

- ½ cup mushroom
- 1 pc pork sausage
- 5 pc ripe tomato
- ½ cup chopped broccoli
- 1 head lettuce
- 1t balsamic vinegar
- 1t hummus

Instructions:

In a pan, fry the sausage using a low heat fire and cook until done. Use a kitchen napkin or paper towel to reduce the oil in it and drain all fat. Use a clean chopping board to cut the sausage. In a small casserole, bring water to boil and add salt to taste. Place veggies in pouch and cook until crisp. Combine all the ingredients and mix in the seasonings in a large bowl.

Nutrition Facts:

Calories: 105.8
Total fat: 5.2 g
Cholesterol: 10.8 mg
Sodium: 223.3 mg
Total carbs: 11.4 g
Dietary fiber: 3.4 g
Protein: 7.1 g

Crawdad Quick Lunch

Ingredients:

- Crayfish or Crawdad Tail Meat, 12 oz
- Margarine, soft, 3 tbsp
- Teriyaki Sauce, 2 tbsp
- Garlic fresh, minced, 1 tbsp
- Soy Sauce, 3 tbsp
- Lemon Juice , 3 tbsp
- Barbecue Sauce, 1 tbsp
- Salt, pepper, red pepper flakes, chili powder to taste.

Instructions:

In a pan, sauté the meat with margarine. Add a little bit of oil to prevent it from burning. Combine all the listed ingredients accordingly. Mix in the seasonings to add extra flavors. You may serve it with rice if desired.

Nutrition Facts:
Calories; 138.9
Total fat: 6.7 g
Cholesterol: 113.1 mg
Sodium: 1229 mg
Total carbs: 3.4 g
Dietary fiber: .1 g
Protein: 15.7 g

Baked Salmon with Brown Rice

Ingredients:
- 30 oz salmon
- 1/2 cup brown rice
- 1/2 of a yellow bell pepper

Instructions:

Grease a rectangular pan with oil. Rub the salmon with salt and pepper to taste before placing in the pan. Top the fish with a bell pepper for extra aroma and nutrients. Bake for 10 - 15 minutes in a microwave. Serve with brown rice.

Nutrition Facts:
Calories: 344.4
Total fat: 7.3 g
Cholesterol: 94.9 mg
Sodium: 128.6 mg
Total carbs: 28.3 g
Dietary fiber: 2.6 g
Protein: 39.7 g

Low Carb Sushi Roll with Cauliflower Rice

Ingredients:
- 1 Cup cauliflower rice
- 2 tablespoons of rice vinegar
- Freshly grated ginger
- 4 nori sheets
- 1 can tuna in brine
- 1 long shallot, sliced thin lengthwise
- Handful of coriander
- Soy sauce for dipping

Instructions:

In a pan, Sauté cauliflower rice until slightly brown. Stir in the rice vinegar and ginger. Mix it well. Set aside. Transfer it to a large bowl and let it cool. Using a bamboo mat spread your nori wrapper. Carefully spread the rice. Top with the remaining ingredients except the wasabi and roll in. Use a sharp knife to cut the rolls and serve it bite size. Serve with soy sauce and wasabi.

Nutrition Facts:
Calories: 294.8
Total fat: 8.8 g
Cholesterol: 4.8 mg
Sodium: 902.1 mg
Total carbs: 49.5 g
Dietary fiber: 10.1 g
Protein: 11.1 g

Tortilla Lunch Pizza

Ingredients:
- Whole wheat tortilla, 1 serving
- 1 large tomato sliced
- Oregano, ground, .5 tbsp.
- 1 oz. grated low fat Cheese
- 5T olive oil

Instructions:

Preheat oven to 350 degrees Fahrenheit. Place tortilla on a pizza plate and use the oil to grease it. Bake for 2 minutes, until slightly brown. Once done, layer tomatoes and other ingredients on top. Bake for another 5 minutes. Serve hot.

Nutrition Facts:
Calories: 315.3
Total fat: 18.1 g
Cholesterol: 19.6 mg
Sodium: 655.8 mg
Total carbs: 30.2 g
Dietary fiber: 6 g
Protein: 12.3 g

Chicken Stir-Fry

Ingredients:

- 3.5 oz. of chicken tenders (breast) thawed and cut into bite size pieces.
- 3/4 cup of frozen broccoli stir-fry
- 3/4 cup sugar snap stir-fry
- spices to taste

Instructions:
Heat the peanut oil in a wok or a large skillet over medium-high heat. Add the garlic and ginger. Cook the chicken. Cook the vegetables. Make the sauce. Return the chicken to the wok. Prepare the rice or noodles. Garnish the stir-fry.

Nutrition Facts:

Calories: 258.5
Total fat: 4.4 g
Cholesterol: 60.4 mg
Sodium: 429.3 mg
Total carbs: 13.5 g
Dietary fiber: 3.6 g
Protein: 32.3 g

DINNER

Crawfish Etouffee

Ingredients:
- 2 cups craw fish tails
- 1/2 cup green onions
- 1/2 cup celery
- 3 small cloves garlic
- 1/4 cup red bell pepper
- 1/4 cup green bell pepper
- 1 can 98% fat free cream of mushroom
- ¼ cup 2% milk
- ¼ cup water
- 1 tablespoon light margarine
- 1/2 teaspoon crab boil
- 4 oz. of fat free cream cheese
- 2 cup brown instant rice
- 48 spears of asparagus
- 1 teaspoon lemon juice
- dash of salt and pepper
- 2 tablespoons blue bonnet light

Instructions:
Sauté veggies in margarine. Add crawfish, cream of mushroom water milk and crab boil. Add cream cheese. Let simmer for about 30 min. Cook rice according to directions. Melt 2 tablespoons margarine then add asparagus, dash of salt/pepper and 1 teaspoon lemon juice. Serves 4- each should get 12 spears asparagus, ½ cup rice, and ½ cup etouffee.

Nutrition Facts:
Calories: 316.3
Total fat: 7.8 g
Cholesterol: 174.5 mg
Sodium: 622.6 mg
Total carbs: 29.8 g
Dietary fiber: 5.7 g
Protein: 30.3 g

Complete Salmon Dinner

Ingredients:

- 40 oz salmon
- ½ cup brown rice
- 1 cup broccoli
- 2 tablespoons cheese
- salt, to taste
- Garlic Powder, to taste
- Onion powder, to taste
- Parsley, to taste
- 1 tablespoon oil

Instructions:

Preheat oven to 350 degrees Fahrenheit. Grease a nonstick pan or a baking tray with oil to prevent the fish from sticking. Season the salmon with all the seasonings listed above. Bake the salmon in the oven for about 10 - 15 minutes. While baking the salmon, in a casserole bring the water to boil and start steaming the broccoli.

Check the salmon, when it is cooked and ready to serve, place rice in bowl and baked salmon on top. Then, top salmon with broccoli. Serve hot.

Nutrition Facts:

Calories: 340
Total fat: 8 g
Cholesterol: 103 mg
Sodium: 268 mg
Total carbs: 32 g
Dietary fiber: 3 g
Protein: 29 g

Slow Cooker Pork Chop Dinner

Ingredients:
- 4 cuts pork chop
- 1 tablespoon olive oil
- 1 medium white or yellow onion, sliced
- 2 cups sliced mushrooms
- 1 tablespoon flour
- 1 1/2 cups unsalted chicken stock
- 2 teaspoons no salt Italian seasoning blend
- 1/4 teaspoon black pepper
- 1 pound redskin potatoes, quartered
- 4 cups fresh green beans, trimmed

Instructions:

In a pan, sauté the pork over a medium-high heat and let it release its natural oil.

When done set aside the pork. Sautee onion using a low heat to avoid over cooking. Mix in the mushroom until cook and tender, stir in the flour for 1 minute and gradually pour in the stock. Combine the potatoes and the pork all together then cover. Cover and cook it using a slow cooker for 5 hours. Serve hot.

Nutrition Facts:
Calories: 418.6
Total fat: 19.8g
Cholesterol: 65 mg
Sodium: 79.5 mg
Total carbs: 37.3 g
Dietary fiber: 6.6 g
Protein: 25.8 g

Portobello Steak Dinner

Ingredients:

- 4 Portobello mushroom caps
- 1 cup chopped onions
- 1 cup chopped sweet red peppers
- 6 tbsps. Balsamic vinegar
- 1 tbsps. Extra virgin olive oil
- 4 slices of prosciutto
- 2 oz. soft goat's cheese
- 1 tsp garlic powder
- 1 tbsps. black pepper
- dash of salt

Instructions:

Using a shallow plate, place the mushroom, garlic and black pepper and mix. Mix in the vinegar gradually and let the mushroom absorb the flavor. Marinate it for 2 hours and put it in the fridge. Meanwhile, sauté the onion in a pan and wait until it caramelizes. Set aside. When you are done with the other procedure, preheats the oven to 350 degrees Fahrenheit. Grease cupcake cup or a muffin pan and pour in mushrooms. Top the mushroom with the sautéed onion and bell pepper. Top with cheese and drizzle with oil. Put a pinch of salt and pepper to taste. Bake for 20 - 25 minutes.

Nutrition Facts:
Calories: 207.7
Total fat: 11.9 g
Cholesterol: 26.5 mg
Sodium: 798.5 mg
Total carbs: 16.6 g
Dietary fiber: 3.5 g
Protein: 11.7 g

Filling and Easy Rice Dinner

Ingredients:
- 3/4 lb. extra lean hamburger
- 4-1/2 cups instant white rice
- 1 can cream of chicken soup
- 1-1/2 cups fresh broccoli
- 1-1/2 cups fresh cauliflower
- 3-3/4 cups water

Instructions:

In a pan, fry the burger patties 2 minutes each side until brown and well done. Using a separate pan, bring water to boil and add in the vegetables. When the vegetables are cook and tender, mix in the diced burger patties and let it simmer for another 5 minutes. Turn off the heat and combine it with rice. The rice will absorb the water, and it will be ready to serve. Serve it hot.

Nutrition Facts:
Calories: 170.5
Total fat: 6.3 g
Cholesterol: 21.5 mg
Sodium: 185.5 mg
Total carbs: 20.1 g
Dietary fiber: 1 g
Protein: 8 g

Slow Cooker Boiled Dinner Combo

Ingredients:

- 4 cups of water
- 1 lean 2 lb. beef roast, corned beef roast or ham
- 2 medium onions peeled and halved
- 4 carrots, peeled and cut in half
- 1/2 a large cabbage cut in 4 wedges
- 1 large turnip, peeled and cut in wedges
- 2 potatoes, peeled and cut in half
- 2 beef flavored Bouillon cubes
- 2 bay leaves
- 2 cloves of garlic
- salt and pepper to taste

Instructions:

In a slow cooker, combine all the ingredients and use the heat to a low heat. Cook for at least 3 - 5 hours in a slow cooker. Serve it hot and with vegetables or fruit juices.

Nutrition Facts:
Calories: 270.3
Total fat: 10.1 g
Cholesterol: 51.4 mg
Sodium: 2791.7 mg
Total carbs: 26.7 g
Dietary fiber: 5 g
Protein; 19.4 g

Yankee Pot Roast Dinner

Ingredients:

- Cooking Spray
- 2 1/2 pound lean beef round, well-trimmed
- 1/2 tsp black pepper
- 1/4 tsp table salt
- 2 large onion sliced
- 1 3/4 cup water
- 1 packet onion soup mix
- 1 1/2 Tbsp. balsamic vinegar
- 1 tsp dried thyme
- 8 medium potato
- 1 pound baby carrots
- 1 Tbsp. parsley, fresh, chopped

Instructions:

Preheats the oven to 350 degrees Fahrenheit. Using a shallow baking rack or tray, lay the beef and season with salt and pepper to taste. Top the beef with the vegetables add water and cook for 5 minutes. When it boils, stir it carefully. Cover with foil and bake for 1 hour. Add in the potato and carrots and the cook for another 30 minutes. Transfer it to a cutting board add a slice to a serving size. Garnish with parsley and pour some gravy on it.

Nutrition Facts:
Calories: 299.5
Total fat: 5.7 g
Cholesterol: 80.8 mg
Sodium: 260.3 mg
Total carbs: 25.1 g
Dietary fiber: 3.6
Protein: 35.2 g

Ham and Green Bean Dinner

Ingredients:
- 2 lb. quarter ham roast
- 6 medium sized potatoes for baking
- 1 12oz can of green beans
- 1 cup of ginger

Instructions:

Preheats the oven to 350 degrees Fahrenheit. Place the ham roast in a baking pan. Grease your baking pan with oil to avoid sticking. Combine with the ginger and potatoes on top. Bake for 20 minutes. Cover the top to avoid burns. When the ham is cooked then adds the beans. Serve hot.

Nutrition Facts:
Calories: 190.7
Total fats: 1.5 g
Cholesterol: 13.3 mg
Sodium: 490.6 mg
Total carbs: 36.4 g
Dietary fiber: 2.3 g
Protein: 8.4 g

Balsamic Black Bean & Rice Dinner

Ingredients:

- 1 serving brown rice
- 1 serving reduced sodium black beans
- 1 oz. diced onion
- 1 oz. diced tomato
- 1 oz. diced green pepper
- 1 c. cauliflower
- 1 c. broccoli
- 1 tbsps. Olive oil
- 1 tbsps. Balsamic vinegar
- 1 tbsps. Cumin
- 1 tbsps. Garlic powder

Instructions:

Using low heat, sauté the vegetables in a pan. Stir in the vinegar and mix thoroughly until cook and tender. When the vegetable is cooked, add in the cooked brown rice. Mix in all the seasoning for the flavors. Serve hot and enjoy.

Nutrition Facts:
Calories: 538.1
Total fat: 16 g
Sodium: 38.8 mg
Total carbs: 86.9 g
Dietary fiber: 16.1 g
Protein: 19.1 g

Salmon and Rice Dinner with Broccoli

Ingredients:
- 3 pc Salmon Fillets
- 1 cup long grain rice, cooked
- 1 cup frozen broccoli
- Lemon and lime juice, kosher salt, dill seasoning

Instructions:

Prepare your grill for this recipe. Rinse the salmon fillet to remove the slimy liquid on it. Rub the salmon with salt and lemon before grilling to taste. Grill over a low heat until tender. Serve with a cup of rice and top with steamed broccoli.

Nutrition Facts:
Calories: 435.4
Total fat: 12.5 g
Cholesterol:' 101 mg
Sodium: 729.3 mg
Total carbs: 33.3 g
Dietary fiber: 5.7 g
Protcin: 42.4 g

SNACKS

Mini Nacho Cups

Ingredients:

- 8 baked scoop-shape tortilla chips
- 2 Tablespoons guacamole
- ¼ cup chopped cherry tomatoes
- 1 tablespoon low fat cheese
- 1 tablespoon thinly sliced green onion

Instructions:

Rinse tomatoes carefully to remove dirt and other contaminants. Slice the onion thinly and set aside. If you want, you can buy some guacamole, or if you prefer you can make it from scratch. In a clean plate, arrange the nacho or tortilla chips and top the tomatoes and onion. Grate the cheese on the top of it. Serve with the guacamole.

Nutrition Facts:
Calories: 132
Total fat: 2 g sat. fat
Cholesterol: 5 g
Sodium: 229 mg
Carbohydrates: 15 g
Fiber: 4g
Sugars: 1g
Protein: 2g

Smoked Salmon Appetizers

Ingredients:

- 3 tablespoons sliced green onions
- 1 1/2 teaspoons finely shredded lemon peel
- 4 teaspoons lemon juice
- 4 teaspoons olive oil
- 4 teaspoons capers
- 1 1/2 teaspoons anchovy paste (optional)
- 2 cloves garlic, minced
- 1/4 teaspoon freshly ground pepper
- 1 4-oz. piece smoked salmon, cut 12- to 1-inch thick
- Olives or olive medley, cut up (about 24 olives)
- Coarsely chopped roasted red sweet peppers
- 6 hard-cooked eggs, cut into 12-inch slices
- Crackers or toasted pita wedges

Instructions:

In a small serving bowl, mix green onion, lemon peel, lemon juice, olive oil, capers, anchovy paste, garlic, and ground pepper. Place the salmon on a serving plate, surrounded with small bowls of olives, roasted red pepper, egg slices, and caper mixture. Serve with crackers and toasted pita wedges.

Nutrition Facts:

Calories: 93
Total fat: 5 g
Cholesterol: 108 mg
 Sodium: 229 mg
Carbohydrates: 15 g
Fiber: 2 g
Sugars: 1 g
Protein: 4 g

Fried Onion Rings

Ingredients:

- Nonstick cooking spray
- 1/4 cup refrigerated or frozen egg product, thawed
- 2 tablespoons buttermilk
- 3/4 cup panko (Japanese-style bread crumbs)
- 1/4 teaspoon Cajun seasoning, blackened seasoning, or barbecue seasoning
- 1 large sweet onion cut into 1/4-inch-thick slices and separated into rings

Instructions:

In a large saucepan, combine cut-up reduced-fat cream cheese; fat-free milk; garlic, minced; and ground black pepper. Cook over a low heat until melted and smooth, when whisking constantly; you can remove it from heat. Then whisk in light dairy sour cream. Add green beans; toss to coat. Then preheat oven to 400 degrees F. Trim haricot vets or tender young green beans. In another large covered saucepan, cook beans in a small amount boiling water for around 8 to 10 minutes; drain and set aside. Spread green bean mixture in a rectangular baking dish. Bake, uncovered, about until heated through, normally 15 minutes, stirring once halfway through baking. Top with half of the Fried Onion Rings before serving.

Nutrition Facts:
Calories: 53
Sodium: 58 mg
Carbohydrates: 10 g
Fiber: 1 g
Sugars: 3 g
Protein: 3 g

Rice Cracker Trail Mix

Ingredients:
- 4 cups assorted rice crackers
- 3/4 cup dried apricots cut into half
- 3/4 cup lightly salted cashews
- 1/4 cup chopped sweetened ginger or raisins

Instructions:

Using a large mixing bowl, combine all ingredients. Use a spatula for better mixing. Serve immediately to enjoy the snack.

Nutrition Facts:
Calories: 102
Total fat: 3 g
Sodium: 78 mg sodium
Carbohydrates: 17 g
Protein: 2 g
Fiber: 1 g

Light 'n Crisp Egg Rolls

Ingredients:

- 2 teaspoons toasted sesame oil or canola oil
- 8 ounces lean pork loin, cut into 1/2-inch pieces, or ground pork
- 1/2 cup chopped red sweet pepper
- 1 teaspoon grated fresh ginger or 1/4 teaspoon ground ginger
- 1 clove garlic, minced
- 3/4 cup finely chopped bok Choy or Chinese cabbage
- 1/2 cup chopped canned water chestnuts
- 1/2 cup coarsely shredded carrot
- 1/4 cup sliced green onions
- 1/4 cup bottled light Asian sesame ginger vinaigrette
- 8 egg roll wrappers

Instructions:

Using a nonstick cooking spray. Preheat oven to 450 degrees Fahrenheit. Line a large baking sheet with foil; lightly coat with nonstick cooking spray; set aside. For filling: In another medium nonstick skillet, heat oil over medium-high heat. Then Add pork, sweet pepper, ginger, and garlic. Cook it for about 3 to 4 minutes or until pork is no longer pink, stirring occasionally. If using ground pork, drain off fat. Add Bok Choy, water chestnuts, carrot, and green onions to pork mixture in skillet. Cook and stir about 1 minute more or until any liquid evaporates. Stir in vinaigrette. Cool filling slightly.

For the assembly, each egg roll is placed in a roll wrapper on a flat surface with a corner pointing toward you. Fold the bottom corner over filling, tucking it under on the other side. Fold side corners over filling, forming an envelope shape. Roll egg roll toward remaining corner. Moisten top corner with water; press firmly to seal.

Place egg rolls, seam sides down, on the prepared baking sheet. Coat the tops and sides of the egg rolls with nonstick cooking spray. Bake for 15 to 18 minutes or until egg rolls is golden brown and crisp. Cool slightly before serving.

Nutrition Facts:

Calories: 167
Total Fat: 4 g
Cholesterol: 22 mg
Sodium: 282 mg
Carbohydrates: 23 g carb
Protein: 10 g
Sugar: 1 g

DESSERTS

Berry Dessert Nachos

Ingredients:
- 3 8 - inches plain or whole wheat flour tortillas
- 1 tablespoon butter, melted
- 2 teaspoons sugar
- 1/8 teaspoon ground cinnamon
- 3/4 cup fat-free or light dairy sour cream
- 3/4 cup frozen light whipped dessert topping, thawed
- 1 teaspoon vanilla
- 1/8 teaspoon ground cinnamon
- 3 cups fresh raspberries and/or blackberries
- 2 tablespoons sliced almonds, toasted
- 1 tablespoon grated semisweet chocolate

Instructions:

Preheat oven to 350 degrees Fahrenheit. In a medium mixing bowl, use spatula to combine the cream, vanilla, and cinnamon. Cover the mixture and put in a fridge.

While cooling the mixture, prepare the tortilla. Spread the tortilla each side with melted butter. In a separate bowl, combine the sugar and cinnamon and sprinkle it over the tortilla. Grease the baking sheets at start baking the tortilla for 5 minutes. When the tortilla is cool and ready to serve, top it with the cream and some berries. For an added kick of flavor, top with grated chocolates and almonds.

Nutrition Facts:
Calories: 213
Total fat: 7 g
Cholesterol: 8 mg
Sodium: 168 mg
Carbohydrates: 31 g carbs
Fiber: 5 g
Protein: 5 g

Frozen Pineapple Dessert

Ingredients:
- 2 cups pineapple chunks, frozen
- 4 teaspoons sugar
- 1 teaspoon fresh lime juice

Instructions:

Using a blender, combine pineapple, sugar, and lime juice. Blend until smooth. If desired, garnish with shredded lime peel. And then you can serve it as fast as that.

Nutrition Facts:
Calories: 55
Sodium: 1 mg
Carbohydrates: 14 g
Fiber: 1 g
Sugar: 12 g

Peach-Berry Frozen Dessert

Ingredients:

- 1 8 - ounce package fat-free cream cheese, softened
- 2 6 - ounce carton peach fat-free yogurt
  with artificial sweetener
- 1/2 8 - ounce container frozen light whipped dessert
  topping, thawed
- 1 cup chopped and peeled fresh peaches; frozen
  unsweetened peach slices, thawed, drained, and
  chopped; or one 8-1/4-ounce can peach slices (juice
  pack), drained and chopped
- 1 cup fresh or frozen unsweetened blueberries,
  raspberries, and/or strawberries, thawed and drained if
  frozen

Instructions:

Using a medium bowl, combine cream cheese and yogurt.
Then beat with an electric mixer on medium speed until
smooth. Next, fold in the whipped topping, peaches, and the 1
cup berries. Then pour into a 2-quart square baking dish.
Lastly, cover with foil and freeze about 8 hours or until firm.
Before serving, let it stand at the room temperature about 45
minutes to thaw slightly. Then cut it into squares. If desired,
garnish with mint leaves and additional berries. It makes nine
servings.

Nutrition Facts:

Calories: 89 cal.
Total fat: 2 g
Cholesterol: 3 mg cholesterol
Sodium: 159 mg
Carbohydrates: 12 g
Fiber: 1 g
Protein: 6 g

Ginger-Berry Dessert

Ingredients:
- 1/4 cup vanilla fat-free Greek yogurt
- 1/4 cup fresh raspberries
- 1 gingersnap cookie, crushed

Instructions:

Using a large mixing bowl, combine all the mentioned ingredients and you will have a quick snack or dessert.

Nutrition Facts:
Calories: 88 cal.
Total fat: 1 g
Sodium: 62 mg
Carbohydrates: 14
Fiber: 2 g
Sugar: 7 g sugars
Protein: 7 g

Melon Dessert Nachos

Ingredients:

- 2 tablespoons sugar
- 1/4 teaspoon ground cinnamon
- 3 6 - 7 - inches whole wheat flour tortillas
- 1/2 cup light tub-style cream cheese, softened
- 1/3 cup light dairy sour cream
- 1 teaspoon finely shredded orange peel
- 1/4 cup orange juice
- 2 cups chopped assorted melon

Instructions:

Preheats the oven to 375 degrees Fahrenheit. Grease the nonstick baking sheet using oil and flour. Using a parchment paper, line the baking sheet and set aside. Mix in the sugar and cinnamon in a small mixing bowl. In a separate bowl, combine all the other ingredients and stir well. Lay the tortilla chips on a baking sheet and top all the other mixture in it. Bake for 15 minutes. In another mixing bowl, mix the melon and the remaining juice. Serve individually with the tortilla and melon mixture.

Nutrition Facts:
Calories: 121 cal.
Total fats: 5 g
Cholesterol: 14 mg
Sodium: 207 mg
Carbohydrates: 18 g
Fiber: 5 g
Protein: 5 g

Improve Your Health with Exercise

In addition to diet, exercise can help you with prevention of diabetes because it not only helps you lose weight and build muscle, it also helps to stabilize your blood glucose levels. Exercise also helps your cells to be more responsive to insulin. You don't have to participate in a marathon in order to get fit. Anything at all that makes you move is considered physical activity. Try accomplishing something that you enjoy such as going for a walk, run, swim, or even gardening- as long as you are moving. Continuous movement will help to burn calories and keep your blood glucose levels right where they need to be.

Even though you may think that you don't have time- the truth is, it really doesn't take that much effort to incorporate some sort of physical activity into your day. At work, instead of taking the elevator, use the stairs- and take a walk around the building or grounds on your lunch break. In the evenings, play a game of catch with your children or go for a walk after dinner. When you're out running errands, park so that you must walk to where you are going.

Aerobics is a great way to start. In fact, some studies are now showing that interval training- that is, alternating between high impact and low impact exercises- is actually the preferred way to control your glucose levels. Why? The reason is that high-intensity interval training, or HIIT, helps to enhance the sensitivity of your liver and adipose tissue to insulin. This means that your muscles also become more receptive to the effects of insulin as they recharge their glucose stores.

However, interval training is not the only way that you can gain control of your blood glucose levels. Resistance training also helps to enhance insulin sensitivity and gain control of blood glucose levels. Still, you're going to burn more calories with resistance training than you are with interval training. This is because strength training requires more muscle- which means that your muscles will require more glucose.

Therefore, when you have been diagnosed with a condition such as insulin resistance or other diabetic condition, exercise should be treated like a physician-prescribed medication. You must always be sure to have the proper dosage on a regular basis. Keep in mind that this is your life we are talking about.

Exercise Tips

Exercising helps you improve your overall health as it allows you to improve your insulin resistance problems. Feeling hungry after your workout? Keep in mind that the rule of "calories in, calories out" does not apply in this situation. Remember always to follow this important tip whenever you feel hungry after exercise: eat proteins with vegetables as well as fats when you feel hungry, then stop eating once you feel full.

There are a lot of exercise routines for you to try as a complement to your insulin resistance diet. Make sure you choose something you actually enjoy doing as this helps you: 1) stick to doing it regularly; 2) try to challenge yourself; and 3) reap its energizing benefits. Just remember to start at a pace that you are comfortable with and consult your doctor before getting started on any exercise routine.

1. Dancing

Dancing allows you to indulge in a fun activity as you move your body, increase your heart rate, cleanse your body from the inside out through perspiration, curb your sugar cravings, and increase your energy levels. Make your dancing routines even more enjoyable by putting on your favorite music.

2. Calisthenics/Bodyweight exercises
Calisthenics is a great way for you to burn fat, increase your flexibility, and improve your energy levels without too much effort and the need for any expensive equipment.

3. Hiking

You can hike anywhere and at your pace to improve your energy levels as well as give your muscles and heart a good challenge. You also get to enjoy the fresh air and pleasant scenery as you do your hiking.

4. Swimming

Swimming is considered one of the most effective exercises you can do to improve your strength as well as your heart health, which contributes to raising your energy levels. Plus, nothing beats swimming as a refreshing workout that lets you burn fat without (literally) sweating it out.

5. Yoga

Yoga may be a relaxing exercise routine, but don't underestimate its ability to raise your energy levels as well. In addition to its being a low-impact activity, what makes yoga such a great exercise is the fact that you can do it in the gym or the comfort of your home. Plus, you can perform it without giving mind to your state of wellness or age.

6. Isometrics

Isometrics is an energizing exercise routine that consists of steps that make you work your muscles against a fixed object (such as planks or walls) or with immovable weights.

7. Plyometrics

Plyometrics (or jump training) consists of exercises that allow you to strengthen your muscles effectively in the hip and leg areas. Plyometrics also allows your body to burn fat efficiently in addition to giving your cardiovascular system a boost.

Seniors are more inclined to creating diabetes, yet a little practice could have a major effect. A study distributed today in Diabetes Care observed that three short strolls every day after suppers were as compelling at decreasing glucose more than 24 hours as a solitary 45-minute stroll at the same moderate pace. Far superior, taking a night established was observed to be significantly more viable at bringing down glucose taking after dinner. The night feast, frequently the biggest of the day can essentially raise 24-hour glucose levels.

Conclusion

Thank you again for purchasing this book!

I hope this book was able to help you understand that just because you have been diagnosed with insulin resistance, you don't have to let that weigh you down. Hopefully this book has been able to set you straight on what insulin resistance is and that it can lead to diabetic conditions such as prediabetes and type 2 diabetes. However, you can get control of it and get to a healthier way of life with lots of energy and a flatter belly as well.

The next step is to educate yourself more on the subject of insulin resistance to enhance your insulin resistance diet. Consider learning more about the glycemic index and how it relates to each food item in your insulin resistance diet menu as well as find ways to make insulin resistance diet-friendly versions of your favorite dishes, beverages, and snacks. Make sure to keep acting on the things you have learned from this book long after you have achieved your desired results. To keep yourself going on the insulin resistance diet, always picture the better version of yourself that the diet has helped you become – lighter, healthier, and more active!

Finally, if you enjoyed this book, then I'd like to ask you for a favor, would you be kind enough to leave a review for this book on Amazon? It'd be greatly appreciated!

Thank you and good luck!

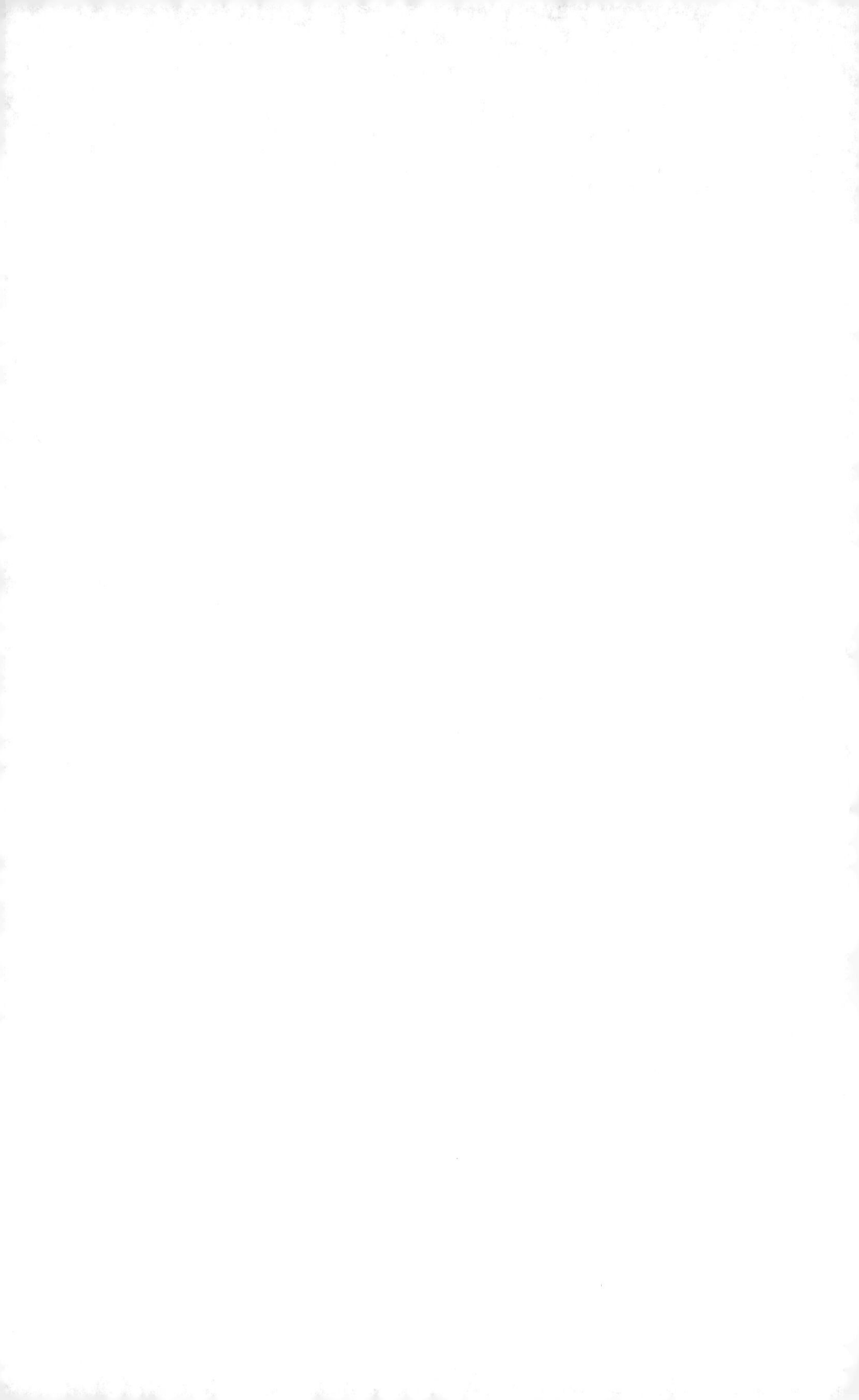

www.ingramcontent.com/pod-product-compliance
Lightning Source LLC
Chambersburg PA
CBHW060642290526
45793CB00001B/354